Healthy Choices

BOOKWORMS

EATING HEALTHY FOODS

By R. J. MacReady

Cavendish Square
New York

Published in 2022 by Cavendish Square Publishing, LLC
243 5th Avenue, Suite 136, New York, NY 10016

First Edition

Library of Congress Cataloging-in-Publication Data

Names: MacReady, R. J., author.
Title: Eating healthy foods / R.J. MacReady.
Description: First edition. | New York : Cavendish Square Publishing, [2022] | Series: Healthy choices | Includes index.
Identifiers: LCCN 2020034871 | ISBN 9781502659644 (library binding) | ISBN 9781502659620 (paperback) | ISBN 9781502659637 (set) | ISBN 9781502659651 (ebook)
Subjects: LCSH: Nutrition–Juvenile literature. | Food–Juvenile literature. | Food habits–Juvenile literature.
Classification: LCC RA784 .M277 2022 | DDC 613.2–dc23
LC record available at https://lccn.loc.gov/2020034871

Editor: Greg Roza
Designer: Andrea Davison-Bartolotta

The photographs in this book are used by permission and through the courtesy of: Cover wavebreakmedia/Shutterstock.com; p. 5 Tom Werner/DigitalVision/Getty Images; p. 7 Stan Dzugan/Moment/Getty Images; p. 9 Enrique Diaz/7cero/Moment/Getty Images; p. 11 MirageC/Moment/Getty Images; p. 13 IGphotography/iStock/Getty Images Plus/Getty Images; p. 15 (main) Claudia Totir/Moment/Getty Images; p. 15 (inset) Todd Gipstein/The Image Bank Unreleased/Getty Images; p. 17 (main) Science Photo Library/Getty Images; p. 17 (inset) kaanates/E+/Getty Images; p. 19 baibaz/iStock/Getty Images Plus/Getty Images; p. 21 Thurtell/E+/Getty Images; p. 23 kali9/E+/Getty Images.

CPSIA compliance information: Batch #CW22CSQ: For further information contact Cavendish Square Publishing LLC, New York, New York, at 1-877-980-4450.

Printed in the United States of America

CONTENTS

Smart Eating

Food is a big part of life! People need to eat to live and grow. Choosing healthy foods to eat is smart. Healthy foods help your body. What are some healthy foods?

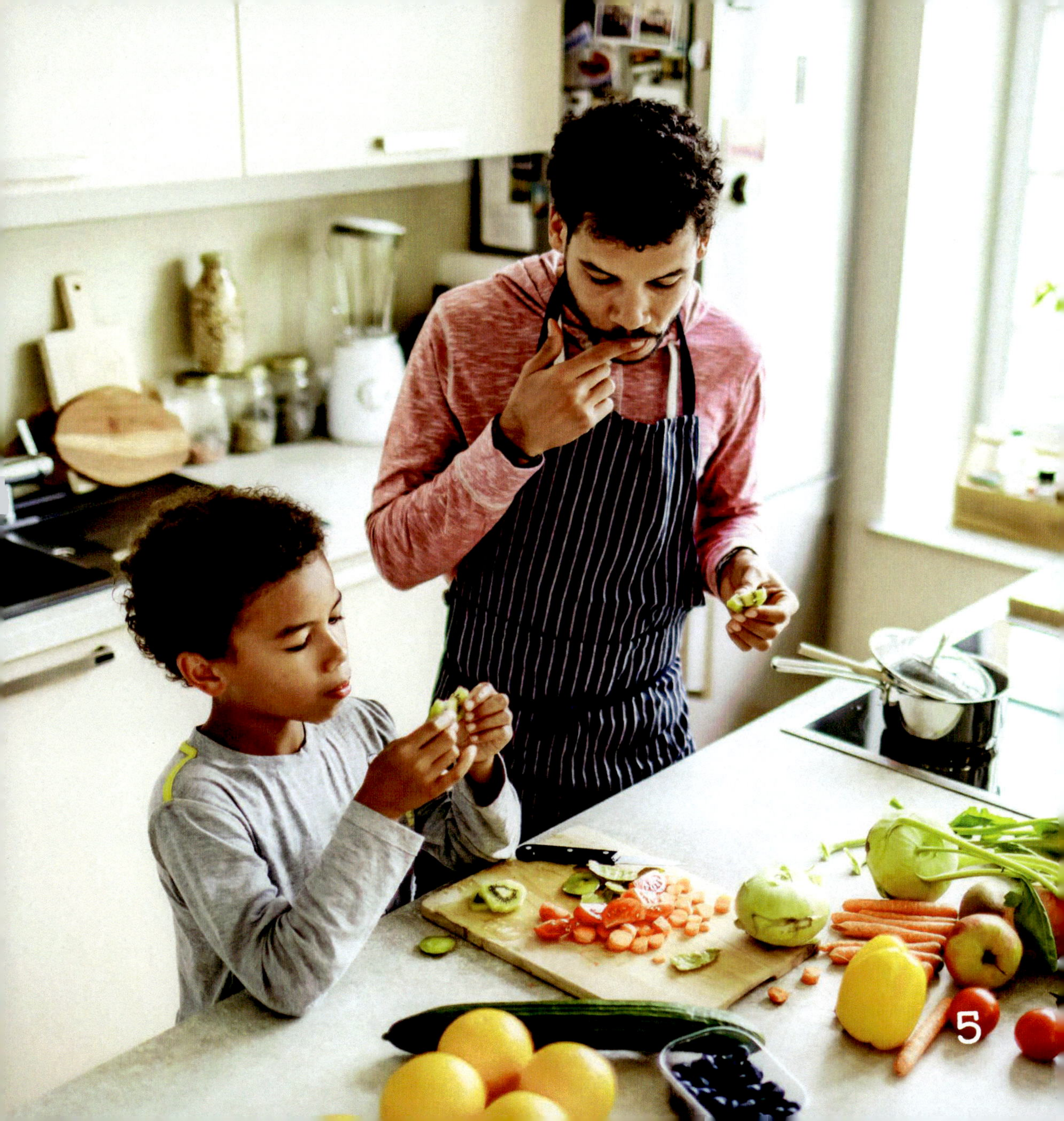

Vegetables are plants or parts of plants. They're filled with healthy **nutrients**. They also have fiber. Fiber helps with **digestion**. It's important to eat different kinds of vegetables every day. They come in many shapes, sizes, and colors!

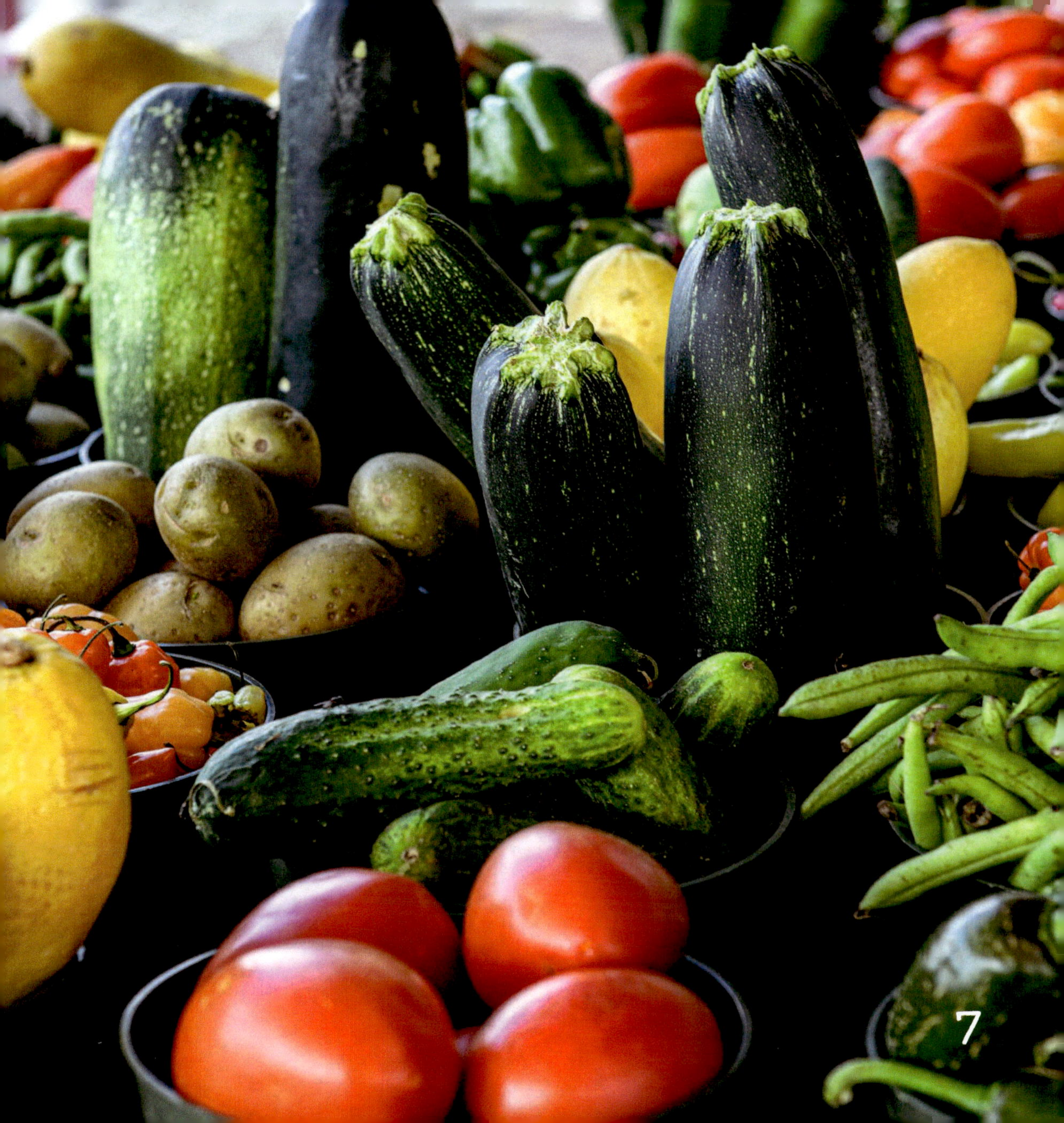

Just like vegetables, fruits come from plants and are filled with nutrients. Most also have fiber. Eating fruit every day can help you stay healthy. Fruits also come in many colors and sizes. It's fun to try new kinds!

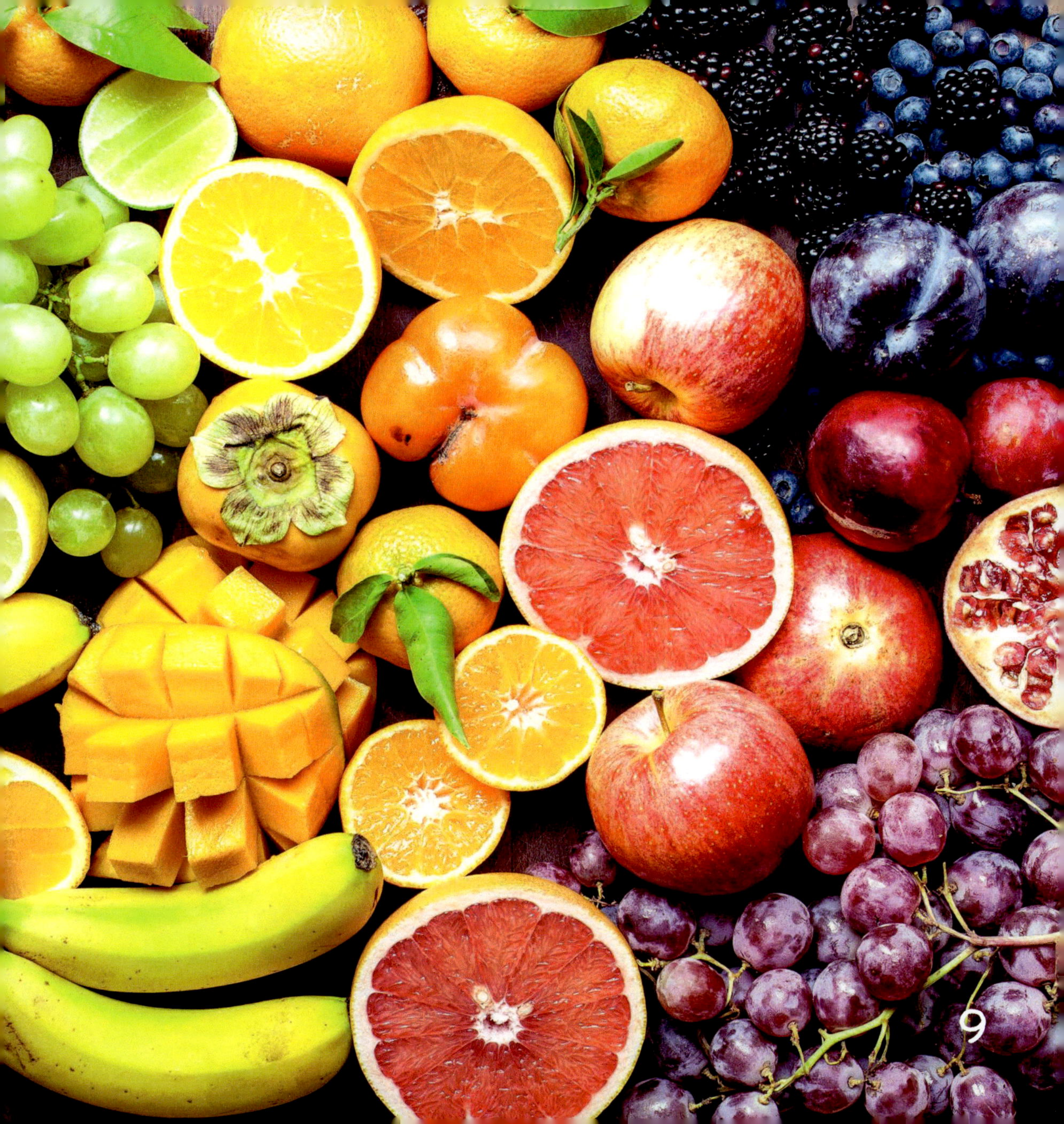

Grains are plants such as wheat, oats, and rice. We use grains to make bread and many other foods. Whole grains are healthier than refined grains. "Refined" means that something is taken out of the grain before it's eaten.

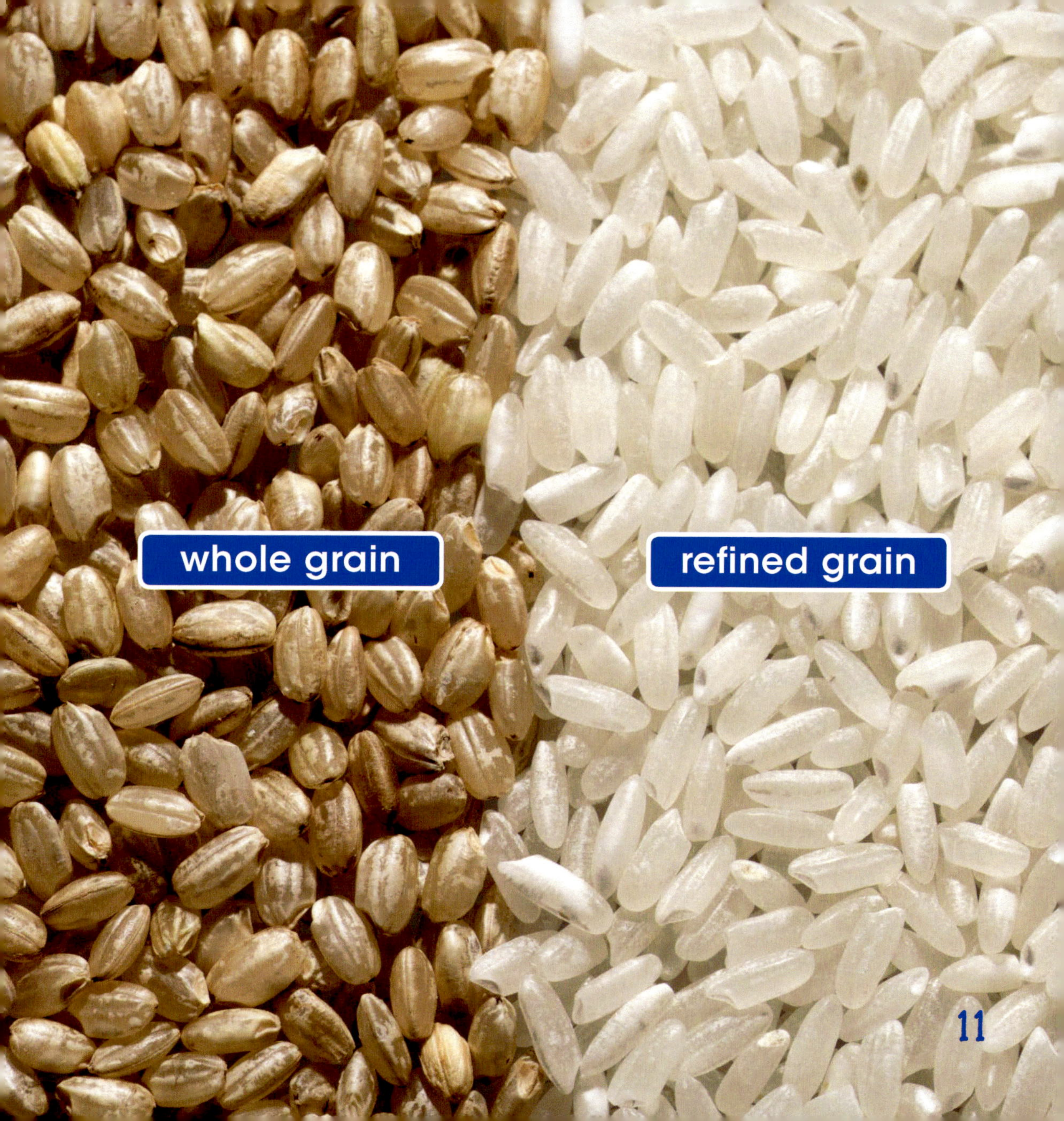
whole grain
refined grain

Making Choices

Our bodies get fats and oils from many foods. We need some fats to have the energy, or power, to work and play. Most healthy fats and oils come from seeds and nuts. Other fats, such as the fats in fried foods, aren't as healthy.

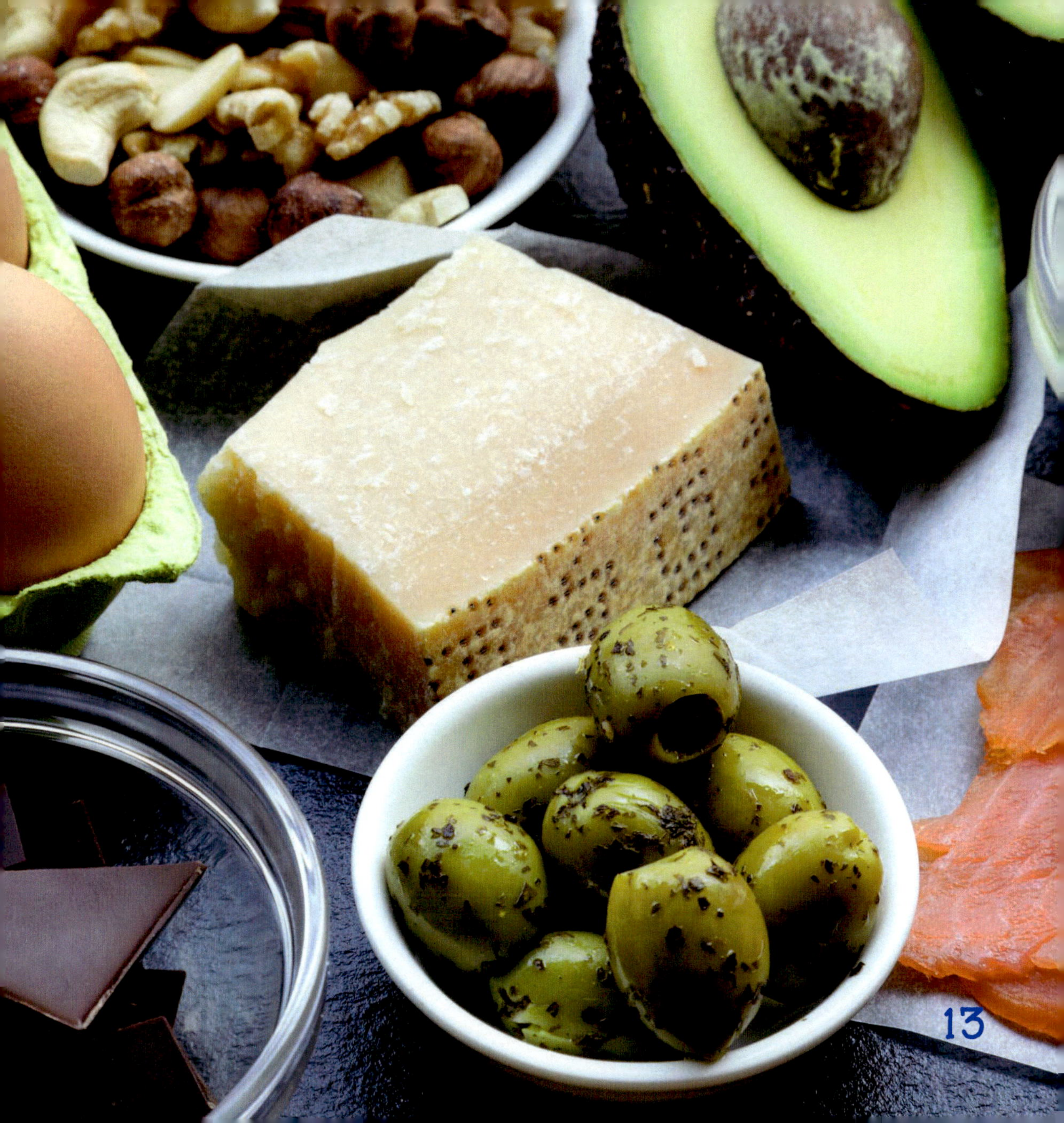

Meats and eggs help the body grow and stay strong. Fish has a lot of healthy fats in it. **Processed** meats are often high in salt and unhealthy fats. It's healthier to eat those kinds of meats less often than fish or chicken.

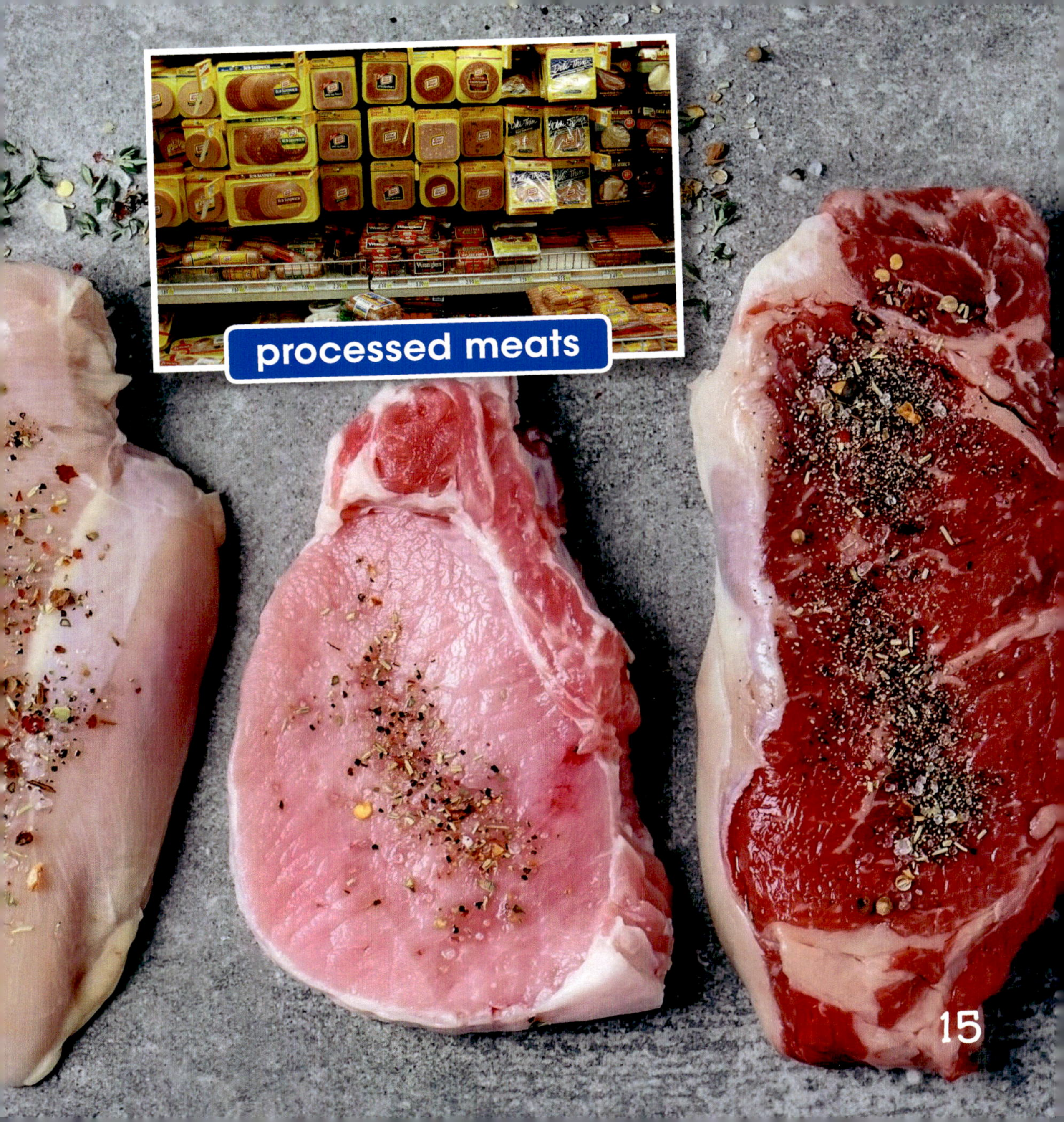

processed meats

Nuts and legumes are high in nutrients and fiber. They can sometimes be eaten instead of meat. The fats and oils in nuts are good for your heart. Legumes include beans, lentils, and peas. They're very healthy foods!

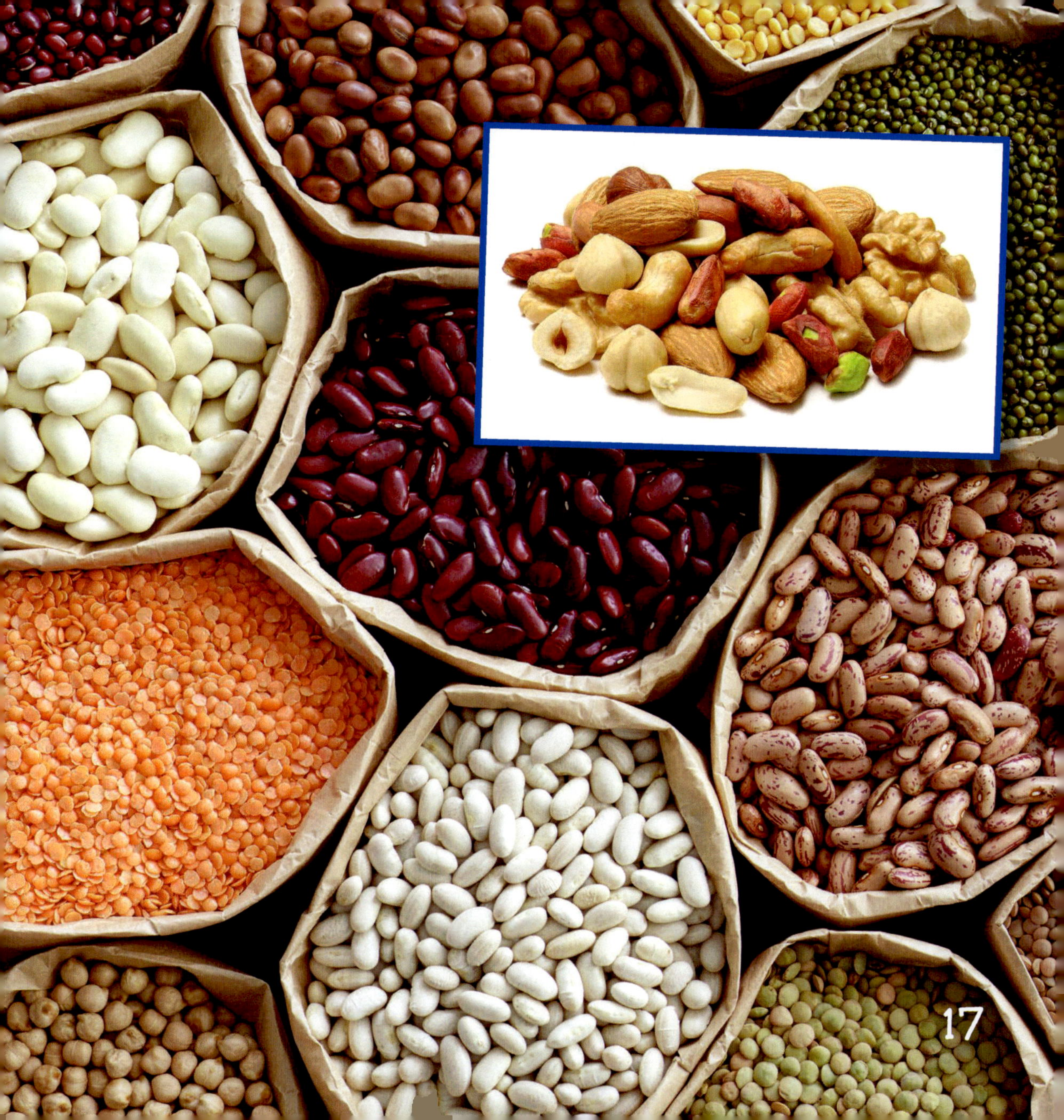

Dairy foods are made from milk. They include cheese and yogurt. Dairy foods have a nutrient that's great for bones and teeth. Adults don't need to eat or drink as much dairy as growing kids.

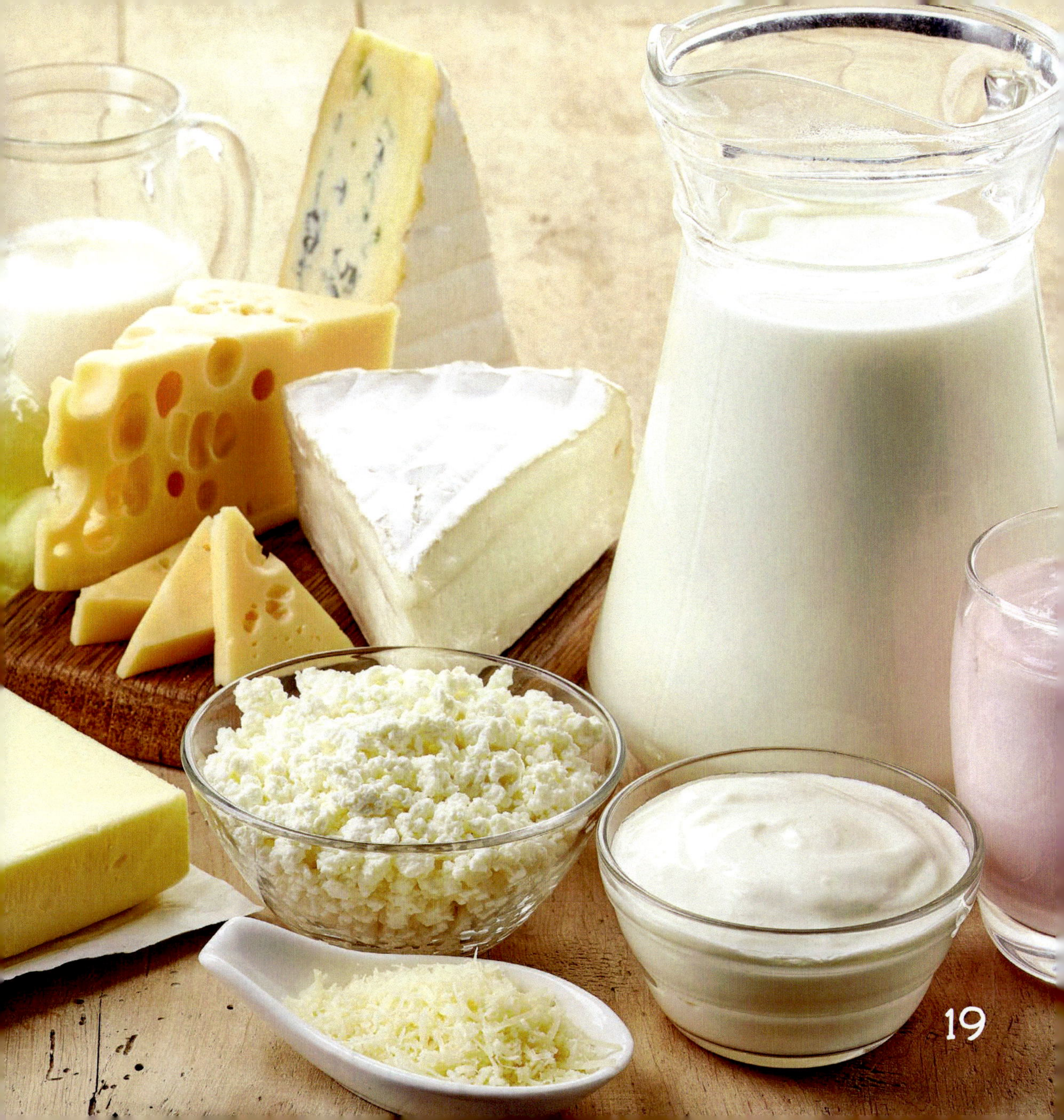

Processed foods have things added to them to make them taste better. Canned and frozen foods often have a lot of salt and sugar. Eating too much salt and sugar isn't healthy. Always read **food labels** to see what's in your food.

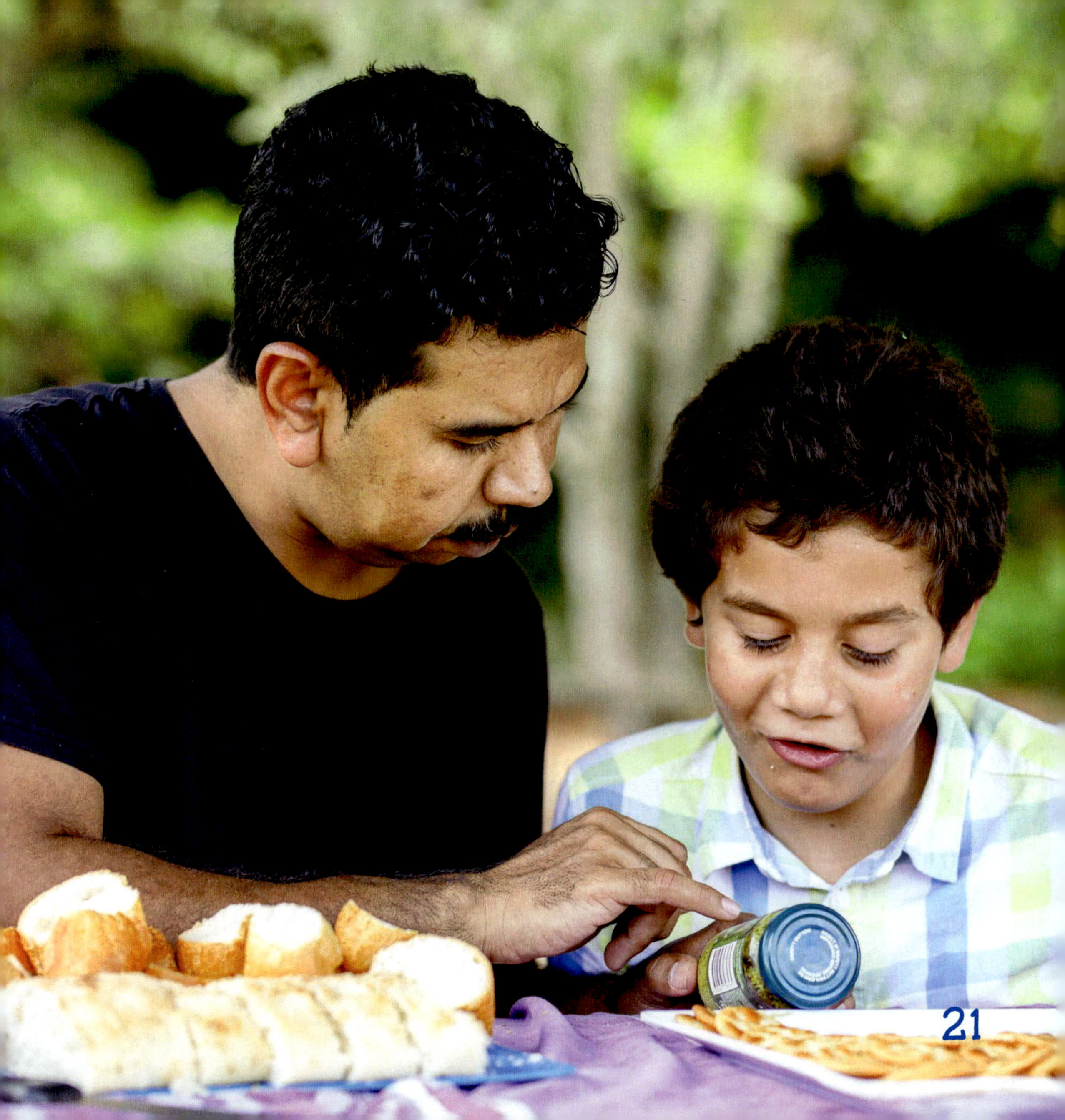

Special Times

Eating healthy foods doesn't mean we have to stop eating things like pizza and cake forever. However, we shouldn't eat them all the time. It's smart to save them for special times—like birthdays!

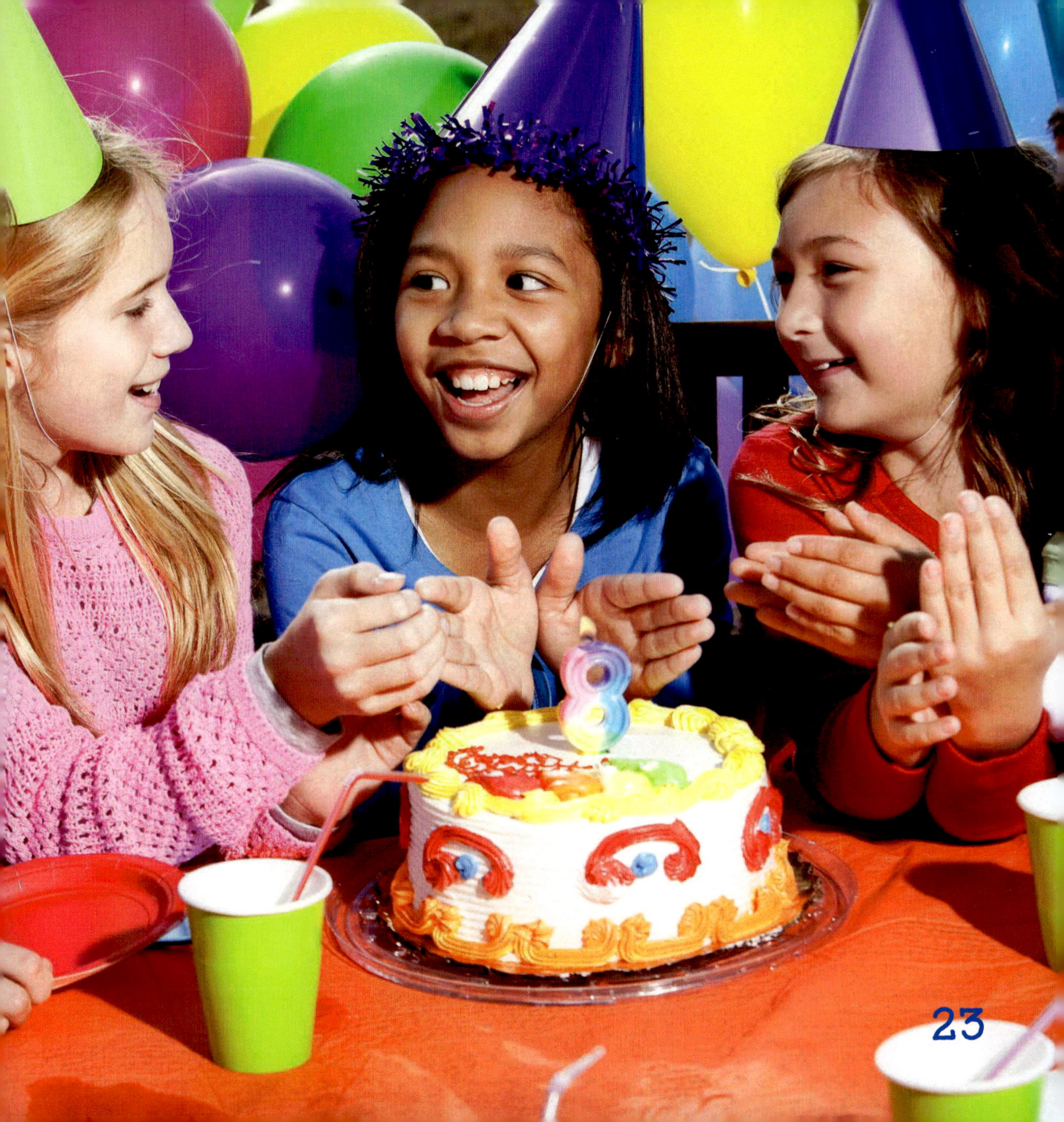

WORDS TO KNOW

digestion: The body's process of breaking food down into nutrients.

food labels: Lists of ingredients and nutrients on foods bought in stores.

nutrients: Natural things in food that the body needs for life and growth.

processed: Having gone through special treatment in a factory.

INDEX